1

Table of Contents

Neutropenic Diet

A low microbial neutropenic diet is essentially a diet that ensures food is safe. Safe means free of microbes such as bacteria, viruses, yeast and molds. To be honest, we all should be preparing our meals so they're safe.

People with healthy immune systems can handle food that has some microbes. Unfortunately, people with weak immune systems cannot. This includes cancer patients who have a low white blood cell count (leukopenia) after undergoing chemotherapy, radiation therapy or a bone marrow or stem cell transplant. People with leukopenia are at a high risk of infection, which is why a doctor might prescribe a low microbial neutropenic diet.

During food preparation, there are several stages where it is important to keep food safe:

- Purchasing ingredients
- Transporting ingredients
- Storing ingredients
- Cleaning the workspace
- Preparing ingredients
- Cooking ingredients
- Storing cooked food

1. **Purchasing Safe Ingredients**

    a. Make sure all items that should be cold stay cold, e.g., dairy products

    b. Buy whole fruits and vegetables (not pre-cut) and make sure they are free of bruises, cuts or mold.

    c. Make sure all bottled/packaged items are properly sealed and have not reached their expiration date.

    d. Buy cheese that is commercially packaged (not cheeses that are cut and rewrapped)

    e. Do not buy from bulk bins, salad bars, deli counters

    f. Keep raw meat/seafood separate (and wrapped properly) from raw produce

g. Buy only pasteurized products, e.g., milk, cheese, juices

h. Do not buy smoked seafood, e.g., lox, smoked salmon

2. Transporting Ingredients Safely

a. Go directly home after purchasing ingredients

b. If it is hot out, bring a cooler/insulated bag with frozen ice packs

3. Storing Ingredients Safely

a. Store ingredients in refrigerator or freezer as soon as you get home

b. Store items on the inside shelves of the refrigerator, not the door

4. Cleaning the Workspace

a. Designate a space in your kitchen for meal preparation

b. Use anti-bacterial cleaning spray and paper towels or a clean cloth to wipe the surface down

c. Use anti-bacterial cleaning spray and paper towels or a clean cloth to clean cutting boards (use plastic cutting board, not wood, and have one cutting board designated for produce and a separate cutting board for raw meats/fish)

5. Preparing Ingredients Safely

a. Wash your hands throughly with soap and water before preparing food and after preparing raw meat/seafood (I like to use disposable food service gloves)

b. Wash produce thoroughly even if you plan on peeling it or cutting it

6. Cooking Ingredient Safely

a. Make sure all foods are completely cooked, including raw fruits and vegetables. Eggs should be hard boiled (unless you use pasteurized eggs, which can be scrambled soft)

b. Well washed thick-skinned fruits can be peeled and eaten, e.g., bananas, avocados, mangos and melons

c. Use a food thermometer to make sure the internal temperature of food reaches the safe minimum temperature

7. Storing Cooked Food Safely

a. Refrigerate food as soon as it is slightly cooled

b. Freeze any food you will not consume within a day or two (freeze individual portions of meatballs, meatloaf and soup in quart-size freezer bags on a baking sheet; this makes for more efficient storage in the freezer. Be sure to label the contents and date)

c. Reheat leftovers to an internal temperature of at least 165 degrees for at least 15 seconds

d. Do not eat food that has been already been reheated once

This diet has been suggested for people living with cancer, as they're more prone to developing bacterial infections. It has also been recommended to people with weakened immune systems — specifically those with neutropenia, whose bodies produce an inadequate amount of white blood cells (neutrophils).

Neutrophils are blood cells that help protect your body from infection. When lower levels of these cells are present, your immune system weakens and your body is less able to defend itself against bacteria, viruses, and infections, including:

- fever

- pneumonia

- sinus infections

- sore throat

- mouth ulcers

Safety Guidelines

Prior to starting the neutropenic diet, discuss your dietary changes and health needs with your doctor to prevent interfering with any treatment plans. In addition, there are some general tips you can pair with the neutropenic diet to safely handle food and help prevent illness.

Some of these guidelines include:

a. Washing your hands before and after handling food, as well as washing all surfaces and utensils

b. Avoiding raw foods, specifically meat and undercooked eggs, along with cooking all meats thoroughly

c. Avoiding salad bars

d. Thoroughly washing fresh fruits and vegetables before eating or peeling (cooked fruits and vegetables are OK to eat)

e. Avoiding unpasteurized dairy products

f. Avoiding well water if it hasn't been filtered or boiled for at least 1 minute (Bottled water is fine if it has been distilled or filtered or undergone reverse osmosis.)

Foods to eat on the Neutropenic Diet

Foods you're allowed to eat on the neutropenic diet include:

1. **Dairy:** all pasteurized milk and dairy products, such as cheese, yogurt, ice cream, and sour cream

2. **Starches:** all breads, cooked pastas, chips, French toast, pancakes, cereal, cooked sweet potatoes, beans, corn, peas, whole grains, and fries

3. **Vegetables:** all cooked or frozen vegetables

4. **Fruits:** all canned and frozen fruit and fruit juices, along with thoroughly washed and peeled thick-skinned fruits like bananas, oranges, and grapefruit

5. **Protein:** thoroughly cooked (well-done) meats and canned meats, as well as hard-cooked or boiled eggs and pasteurized egg substitutes

6. **Beverages:** all tap, bottled, or distilled water, as well as canned or bottled drinks, individually canned sodas, and instant or brewed tea and coffee

Foods to avoid

Foods you should eliminate while following the neutropenic diet include:

1. **Dairy:** unpasteurized milk and yogurt, yogurt made with live or active cultures, soft cheeses (Brie, feta, sharp Cheddar), cheeses with mold (Gorgonzola, blue cheese), aged cheeses, cheeses with uncooked vegetables, and Mexican-style cheeses like queso

2. **Raw starches:** bread with raw nuts, uncooked pasta, raw oats, and raw grains

3. **Vegetables:** raw vegetables, salads, uncooked herbs and spices, and fresh sauerkraut

4. **Fruits:** unwashed raw fruits, unpasteurized fruit juices, and dried fruits

5. **Protein:** raw or undercooked meat, deli meats, sushi, cold meat, and undercooked eggs with runny yolk

6. **Beverages:** sun tea, cold brewed tea, eggnog made with raw eggs, fresh apple cider, and homemade lemonade

Meal Recipes to adopt on the Neutropenic Diet

Baked French Toast

Baked French toast is a fun way to get your carbohydrate fix when you're on a low-fiber diet since it's made without whole grains. The version shown here is a bit like bread pudding in consistency, but you can keep it in the oven longer for a crispier texture. Top with a dollop of ricotta whipped cream if you're feeling decadent.

Prep Time: 10 minutes | Yield: Serves 8

Ingredients

- 2 tablespoons butter or coconut oil, melted
- 6 eggs

- 1½ cups whole milk

- 2 cups whole-milk ricotta cheese

- 1 tablespoon vanilla extract

- ½ teaspoon salt

- 1 loaf bread, sliced (baguette, white bread, Brioche, or challah)

- ¾ cup apricot or peach preserves, or apple jelly

- ¼ cup heavy cream

- 1 tablespoon powdered sugar (optional)

- Maple syrup

Instructions

1. Coat a 9-by-13 baking dish with melted butter.

2. In a large bowl, beat eggs, milk, 1 cup ricotta, vanilla, and salt with a whisk or electric beater.

3. Spread each piece of bread with preserves. Arrange bread in two layers, jam-side up, in prepared baking dish. Pour wet ingredients over bread. Cover with plastic wrap or lid and refrigerate overnight.

4. Preheat oven to 350 degrees. Bake French toast for 45 minutes for a softer, bread-pudding-like texture or for 1-hour for a firmer, crisper texture. If the top begins browning too quickly, loosely cover with aluminum foil. French toast should register 160 degrees Fahrenheit or higher using an

instant-read thermometer placed in the middle of the dish.

5. While French toast is baking, whip cream in a large bowl with an electric beater until stiff peaks form. Gently fold in remaining 1 cup ricotta and powdered sugar, if desired.

6. Serve French toast warm with whipped ricotta cream and maple syrup.

Nutritional Information

Calories: 480 calories, Carbohydrates: 60g, Fat: 17g, Fiber: 2g, Protein: 20g, Saturated Fat: 10g, Sodium: 520mg, Sugar: 22g

Yogurt Parfait with Banana, Peanut Butter, and Corn Flakes

This parfait not only works well with many different diet types, it's loaded with 33 grams of protein. Be sure to leave out the corn flakes if you're experiencing difficulties swallowing.

Prep Time: 10 minutes | Yield: Serves 1

Ingredients

- 2 tablespoons natural creamy peanut butter
- 1 cup low-fat plain Greek yogurt
- ½ medium banana, sliced
- ¼ cup corn flakes cereal

Instructions

1. In a small microwave-safe dish, microwave peanut butter until thin and easy to pour, about 10 to 20 seconds.

2. Spoon ½ cup yogurt into a bowl or air-tight container. Arrange half of the sliced banana over yogurt. Drizzle half of the melted peanut butter over banana. Sprinkle 2 tablespoons cereal over peanut butter. Layer remaining yogurt, banana, peanut butter, and cereal.

3. Serve immediately or chill. Parfait can be stored in an air-tight container up to three days in the refrigerator.

Nutritional Information

Calories: 450 calories, Carbohydrates: 36g, Fat: 21g, Fiber: 4g, Protein: 33g, Saturated Fat: 6g, Sodium: 300mg, Sugar: 23g

Barley Risotto with Butternut Squash

Barley makes for a heartier and nutrient-rich take on the classic risotto made with Arborio rice. You can add well-cooked chicken if you like, or for a vegetarian version, try cannellini beans or tofu.

Prep Time: 65 minutes | Yield: Serves 2

Ingredients

- 2 tablespoons plus 2 teaspoons olive oil

- 1 shallot, finely minced

- ½ cup dry barley

- 3 cups low-sodium vegetable or chicken stock

- 2 cups peeled and diced butternut squash

- ½ teaspoon salt

- ¼ cup crumbled pasteurized milk feta cheese (optional)

Instructions

1. Thoroughly rinse fresh produce under warm running water for 20 seconds. Scrub to remove excess dirt.

2. Heat 2 tablespoons olive oil over medium-low heat in a medium saucepan. Add shallot

and cook until softened, 3 to 5 minutes. Add barley and stir well to combine so each kernel is coated.

3. Increase heat to medium high and toast barley, stirring constantly, for 3 minutes. Add 2 tablespoons stock and stir. Continue to add stock, ¼ cup at a time, while continuing to stir, allowing stock to absorb into barley. Continue adding stock until barley is tender, about 30 minutes.

4. While barley is cooking, heat remaining 2 teaspoons olive oil in a small pan. Add butternut squash and salt and cook over low heat until tender and cooked through, about 15 minutes.

5. When barley is tender and most of the stock has been absorbed, add cooked butternut squash and stir well to combine. Add feta, if desired.

6. To serve, risotto should register 145 degrees Fahrenheit or higher on an instant-read thermometer placed in the middle of the dish. Refrigerate risotto within one hour of cooking and eat any leftovers within 48 hours.

Note: Nutrition information does not include the addition of feta cheese.

Nutritional Information

Calories: 430 calories, Carbohydrates: 60g, Fat: 19g, Fiber: 11g, Protein: 6g, Saturated Fat: 3g, Sodium: 800mg, Sugar: 5g

Simple Buttered Noodles with Herbs

The fresh flavor of the parsley takes this dish to the next level.

There are few dishes as simple and comforting as pasta with butter and cheese. It's a great option when you're coping with digestive problems. If you're having trouble swallowing, try a small-shaped pasta, such as pastina or macaroni.

Prep Time: 20 minutes | Yield: Serves 8

Ingredients

- 16 ounces fettuccine or egg noodles
- ½ cup butter
- ⅓ cup reduced-fat Parmesan cheese (or ⅓ cup cottage cheese)
- 1 tablespoon chopped fresh parsley
- Salt and pepper

Instructions

1. Thoroughly rinse fresh produce under warm running water for 20 seconds. Scrub to remove excess dirt, then set aside.
2. Fill a large pot with lightly salted water and bring to a rolling boil. Cook pasta according

to package directions. Drain and return pasta to pot.

3. Add butter, Parmesan cheese, parsley, and salt and pepper to taste. Mix until well combined.

Nutritional Information

Calories: 270 calories, Carbohydrates: 42g, Fat: 7g, Fiber: 2g, Protein: 8g, Sodium: 85mg, Sugar: 3g

Quinoa Salad with Feta

This zesty, versatile dish can be served as a side, appetizer, or even the base of a hearty salad.

Prep time: 35 minutes | Yield: Serves 8

Ingredients

- 2 cups quinoa

- 3½ cups low-sodium chicken or vegetable broth

- 1 cup grape tomatoes, halved

- ⅔ cup chopped fresh parsley

- ½ cup diced cucumber, peeled and seeded

- ½ cup minced red onions

- 4 ounces feta cheese, crumbled

- 3 tablespoons olive oil

- 3 tablespoons red wine vinegar

- 2 cloves garlic, minced

- Juice of 1 lemon

- Salt and pepper

Instructions

1. Thoroughly rinse fresh produce under warm running water for 20 seconds. Scrub to remove excess dirt.

2. Rinse quinoa in a fine-mesh colander under running water for at least 30 seconds. Drain well.

3. In a saucepan, bring rinsed quinoa and broth to a boil. Reduce heat to medium-low, cover, and simmer until quinoa is tender and broth is absorbed, 15 to 20 minutes. Transfer to a large bowl and set aside to cool.

4. Add tomatoes, parsley, cucumber, onions, feta, olive oil, vinegar, and garlic to cooled quinoa and mix to combine. Pour lemon juice over quinoa salad and season with salt and pepper to taste. Toss to coat and refrigerate until ready to serve.

5. Washing the quinoa well before cooking helps to remove bitterness caused by naturally occurring saponins. Saponins are chemical compounds found in quinoa and other plant-based foods, and have been shown to possess a number of health benefits.

Nutritional Information

Calories: 260 calories, Carbohydrates: 31g, Fat: 11g, Fiber: 4g, Protein: 9g, Saturated Fat: 3g, Sodium: 260mg, Sugar: 4g

Baked Sweet Potato hash with Egg

This healthy, satisfying dish works well for a number of special diets. Enjoy it with family or friends over brunch.

Prep time: 35 minutes | Yield: Serves 4-6

Ingredients

- 2 tablespoons olive oil
- 4 sweet potatoes, peeled and shredded

- 1 bunch kale, chopped

- Salt and pepper

- Cooking spray

- 6 eggs

Instructions

1. Thoroughly rinse fresh produce under warm running water for 20 seconds. Scrub to remove excess dirt.

2. Preheat oven to 350 degrees.

3. Heat a large skillet over high heat. Add olive oil and shredded sweet potato and cook until soft, about 10 minutes. Add kale and cook until wilted. Season mixture with salt and pepper to taste.

4. Coat a 9x13 baking dish with cooking spray. Spoon sweet potato mixture into prepared dish. Then, using a spoon, make 6 wells in the mixture, spaced evenly around the dish, and crack an egg into each one. Top with a sprinkle of salt and pepper.

5. Bake until eggs are cooked and yolks are set. Internal temperature of the hash should be 160 degrees using an instant-read thermometer. Serve immediately.

Nutritional Information

Calories: 210 calories, Carbohydrates: 17g, Fat: 12g, Fiber: 3g, Protein: 8g, Saturated Fat: 2.5g, Sodium: 290mg, Sugar: 9g

Pasta with Kale and Black Olives

This recipe is super fast, super easy and super tasty neutropenic option. You can have it on the table by the time the pasta cooks. Don't hesitate to use pre-cut the kale, or for even less work, frozen.

Prep time: 25 minutes | Serves: 4

Ingredients

- 3 quarts water in a large pot
- 1 tablespoon salt
- 8 ounces whole-wheat pasta, penne, rigatoni
- 3 cloves garlic, smashed and sliced
- 1 whole dried cayenne pepper (optional)

- 1 medium shallot peeled and thinly sliced

- ½ teaspoon sweet smoked paprika

- 1 (2-inch) strip lemon peel, julienned

- 1 x10 ounce pack of frozen kale or 1 bunch Lacinato or Dinosaur kale, steamed (see Ann's Tips)

- 1 (14 ounce) can diced tomatoes, chopped (See Ann's Tips)

- 10-12 oil-cured black olives

- 1 cup pasta water

- 2 tablespoons freshly grated Parmesan cheese

- ½ cup Italian parsley, chopped

- 1 small sprig rosemary, leaves stripped and chopped

- Sea salt and freshly ground black pepper to taste.

Instructions

1. In a large pot add 1 tablespoon of salt to the water and bring to a boil for the pasta.

2. Add the pasta to the boiling water. Cook one minute less than the packet time, approximately 10 minutes for penne or rigatoni. When the pasta is ready, drain reserving a cup of the cooking water. Set aside.

3. Meanwhile, heat the oil in a sauté pan over a medium-high heat. Add the garlic and whole dried red pepper and cook until the

garlic starts to turn light golden about 2 minutes. Add shallots, sprinkle with salt, and cook until they soften and start to color about 5 minutes. Add smoked paprika and lemon peel, stir to coat, then add the steamed or frozen kale and cook, stirring until well mixed.

4. Add the chopped tomatoes and the olives. Cook over a medium heat until the tomatoes look orangey and saucy, about 5-7 minutes. Add ¼ cup water from the pasta pot and stir to mix. Add the grated Parmesan cheese. Cook stirring until it melts into the sauce and the extra water has almost evaporated, about 2 minutes. Do not add salt without

tasting — the olives will have added quite a bit.

5. Stir in the parsley and rosemary. Add the cooked pasta and another ¼ cup of the reserved water. Cook, stirring, until the pasta is just al dente. Serve immediately with freshly grated Parmesan cheese.

Recipe Note

1. If you can't find Lacinato or Dinosaur kale, use regular curly kale prepped as in the Steaming and Freezing Greens recipe.

2. In the summertime, when tomatoes are good use 2 cups chopped ripe beefsteak or Roma tomatoes.

Fusilli with Cream Cheese Pesto Pasta

This creamy pasta dish calls for fusilli and nutrient-rich pesto. If you have difficulties swallowing, use a finer pasta such as pastina or elbow macaroni.

Prep time: 35 minutes | Yield: Serves 4

Ingredients

- 2 cups fusilli
- 6 tablespoons cream cheese, softened
- 3 to 4 tablespoons pesto sauce
- ¼ cup grated Parmesan

45

- Fresh parsley, chopped

- Roasted sunflower seeds

Instructions

1. Cook pasta according to package directions. Reserve about ½ cup cooking liquid, then drain.

2. Whisk cream cheese with pesto and about 6 tablespoons reserved cooking liquid until creamy. Adding more water will produce thinner sauce and less water will produce thicker sauce. Pour sauce over pasta and toss to combine.

3. Top with Parmesan. Add parsley and sunflower seeds to taste, and serve

immediately. Pasta should register 145 degrees Fahrenheit or higher using an instant-read thermometer placed in the middle of the dish.

Nutritional Information

Calories: 320 calories, Carbohydrates: 27g, Fat: 18g, Fiber: 1g, Saturated Fat: 8g, Sodium: 450mg, Sugar: 1g

Cranberry-Stuffed Chicken Breasts

This tart and tangy chicken dish is full of healthy protein without being short on flavor.

Prep time: 45 minutes | Yield: Serves 4

Ingredients

- 1½ tablespoons plus 1 teaspoon olive oil

- 1 small apple, peeled and diced

- ½ cup dried cranberries

- 1 shallot, peeled and diced

- ¾ cup low-sodium chicken stock

- 4 boneless, skinless chicken breasts, about 4 to 6 ounces each

- ¼ cup balsamic vinegar

- Salt and pepper

Instructions

1. Heat 1 teaspoon olive oil in a skillet over medium-high heat. Add apple and cook until tender, 3 to 4 minutes.

2. In a small bowl, combine cooked apple, cranberries, shallot, and 1 tablespoon chicken stock. Set aside.

3. Cut a deep horizontal pocket in the side of each chicken breast. Make the pocket as large as you can without piercing the top or bottom of the breast. Divide apple mixture evenly among chicken breasts, stuffing into each pocket. Secure pockets with toothpicks, threading along the side to close.

4. Heat remaining 1½ tablespoons olive oil in a heavy skillet. Cook chicken, turning once, until golden brown. Add vinegar and remaining chicken stock, then bring to a boil. Lower heat and gently simmer chicken, turning once, 2 or 3 minutes per side.

5. When chicken registers 165 degrees Fahrenheit or higher using an instant-read thermometer placed in the thickest part of the breast, remove from skillet and keep warm.

6. Continue cooking sauce until reduced to a thick syrup. Season with salt and pepper to taste.

7. Spoon sauce over chicken to serve.

Nutritional Information

Calories: 300 calories, Carbohydrates: 20g, Fat: 10g, Fiber: 1g, Protein: 30g, Saturated Fat: 2g, Sodium: 140mg, Sugar: 18g

Lime and Coconut Chicken Breast

The whole family will enjoy these flavorful chicken breasts, which are low in calories and fiber. Marinate ahead of time and you will need only a few minutes to cook the chicken on the stovetop.

Prep time: 45 minutes | Yield: Serves 4

Ingredients

- 2 pounds boneless, skinless chicken breasts

- 1 lime

- 3 tablespoons vegetable oil

- ½ cup coconut milk

- 2 tablespoons low-sodium soy sauce

- 2 tablespoons sugar

- 2 teaspoons curry powder

- 1½ teaspoons ground coriander

- 1 teaspoon ground cumin

- 1½ teaspoons salt

- 4 tablespoons chopped fresh cilantro

Instructions

1. Using a meat tenderizer, pound chicken breasts between sheets of wax paper until ⅛-inch thick.

2. Zest lime into a large bowl; slice lime into wedges and set aside.

3. Add oil, coconut milk, soy sauce, sugar, curry, coriander, cumin, and salt to zest and whisk to combine. Add chicken and toss to combine. Cover and refrigerate for 1 to 2 hours.

4. Remove chicken, reserving marinade. Using a hot sauté pan, grill pan, or cast-iron skillet, brown chicken on both sides. Chicken should register 165 degrees Fahrenheit using an instant-read thermometer inserted in the thickest part of the breast.

5. Meanwhile, pour reserved marinade into a saucepan and bring to a boil. Reduce heat

and simmer for 2 minutes, stirring to prevent burning.

6. Serve sauce over chicken with cilantro and reserved lime wedges.

Nutritional Information

Calories: 330 calories, Carbohydrates: 10g, Fat: 20g, Fiber: 1g, Protein: 28g, Saturated Fat: 7g, Sodium: 1,370mg, Sugar: 7g

Chicken marinated in lemon

You don't need expensive ingredients to prepare a flavorful and delicious chicken dish. The trick is to marinate the chicken ahead of time so that the lemon and spices infuse the meat. Serve with pasta, rice, or cauliflower rice.

Prep time: 25 minutes | Marinade time: 30 minutes – 8 hours | Yield: Serves 4-6

Ingredients

- Juice of 2 lemons
- 2 tablespoons extra-virgin olive oil
- 2 teaspoons lemon pepper
- 1 teaspoon dried basil
- 1 teaspoon dried oregano
- ¼ teaspoon salt
- 4 boneless, skinless chicken breasts

- 4 tablespoons fresh parsley, chopped (optional)
- 4 lemon slices (optional)

Instructions

1. Combine lemon juice, olive oil, lemon pepper, basil, oregano, and salt in a resealable gallon-size plastic bag. Add chicken breasts to bag and shake to coat. Marinate in the fridge at least 30 minutes and up to 8 hours.

2. Heat a heavy skillet over medium-high heat. Add chicken to skillet; discard marinade. Cook 6 to 7 minutes on each side.

Temperature of chicken should be 165 degrees using an instant-read thermometer.

3. Garnish with parsley and lemon slices, if desired.

Nutritional Information

Calories: 350 calories, Carbohydrates: 2g, Fat: 13g, Fiber:0g, Protein: 53g, Saturated Fat: 2.5g, Sodium: 360mg, Sugar: 1g

Butternut Squash and Apple Soup

This creamy, easy-to-swallow soup makes for the ultimate heart-healthy comfort food. The extra depth of flavor comes from roasting the squash and then letting the soup simmer for 30 minutes after blending.

Prep time: 70 minutes | Yield: Serves 12

Ingredients

- 2½ cups butternut squash, peeled and cubed
- 4 tablespoons extra-virgin olive oil
- 1 yellow onion, chopped
- 1 clove garlic, minced
- 5 cups low-sodium vegetable stock
- 2 cups water
- 1 16-ounce can pumpkin puree
- 2 medium red apples, peeled and chopped

- ¼ teaspoon ground cinnamon

- ¼ teaspoon ground nutmeg

- ¼ teaspoon ground cloves

- ¼ teaspoon salt

- ½ teaspoon black pepper

- 4 tablespoons low-fat plain Greek yogurt

- Roasted pumpkin seeds (optional)

Instructions

1. Thoroughly rinse fresh produce under warm running water for 20 seconds. Scrub to remove excess dirt.

2. Preheat oven to 350 degrees.

3. Line a rimmed baking sheet with parchment paper, then spread squash evenly on paper. Drizzle squash with 2 tablespoons olive oil and roast 8 to 10 minutes. Remove from oven and set aside.

4. Heat remaining 2 tablespoons olive oil in a large pot over medium heat. Add onion and garlic. Cook until onion is soft and starts to brown. Add roasted squash, vegetable stock, water, pumpkin puree, apples, cinnamon, nutmeg, cloves, salt, and black pepper. Bring to a boil over high heat, then reduce to a simmer and cook until squash and apples are tender, about 20 minutes. Remove from heat and let cool.

5. Puree soup using an immersion blender, food mill, food processor, or blender. Place pot over low heat until soup is warmed through, about 30 minutes. Add yogurt, stirring until completely combined. Soup should be 145 degrees using an instant-read thermometer.

6. Ladle soup into bowls and garnish with seeds, if using.

Nutritional Information

Calories: 100 calories, Carbohydrates: 14g, Fat: 5g, Fiber: 3g, Protein: 2g, Saturated Fat: 0.5g, Sodium: 65mg, Sugar: 7g

Baked Buffalo Cauliflower Bites

This delicious, easy-to-make snack is a family favorite. It's also low in calories, since the cauliflower is baked instead of fried. Brown rice flour or chickpea flour coat the cauliflower; both ingredients are higher in fiber than all-purpose flour, helping you feel full longer, and higher in protein too.

Prep time: 50 minutes | Yield: Serves 4-6

Ingredients

- Cooking spray
- 2 medium heads cauliflower, cut into small florets

- 1 cup brown rice flour, chickpea flour, or any flour available
- 1 cup water
- 2 teaspoons garlic powder
- 1 teaspoon salt
- 2 teaspoons butter
- 1 ⅓ cups Frank's Hot Sauce

Instructions

1. Thoroughly rinse fresh produce under warm running water for 20 seconds. Scrub to remove excess dirt.

2. Preheat oven to 450 degrees. Line a rimmed baking sheet with parchment paper or spray with cooking spray.

3. Toss the cauliflower florets with flour, water, garlic powder, and salt. Place on prepared baking sheet and bake 20 minutes.

4. In a small saucepan, melt butter with hot sauce. Pour butter mixture over baked cauliflower and toss to coat.

5. Return cauliflower to oven and bake another 20 minutes. Internal temperature of cauliflower should be 145 degrees using an instant-read thermometer. Serve warm.

Nutritional Information

Calories: 130 calories, Carbohydrates: 20g, Fat: 3g, Fiber: 7g, Protein: 7g, Saturated Fat: 1g, Sodium: 1,780mg, Sugar: 5g

Herbed Avocado Egg Salad with Greek Yogurt

Replace the mayonnaise with avocado and creamy non-fat Greek yogurt and you have an egg salad that is heart healthy and safe for people following a low-fiber diet. Top on a slide of bread or serve with salad greens.

Prep time: 25 minutes | Yield: Serves 6

Ingredients

- 10 eggs

- 1 avocado

- ½ cup nonfat plain Greek yogurt

- ½ teaspoon Dijon mustard

- Juice of 1 lemon

- 1 tablespoon chopped chives

- 1 tablespoon chopped dill

- Salt and pepper

- 1 tablespoon olive oil

Instructions

1. Place eggs in a saucepan and fill with water so eggs are covered. Bring to a boil, then

remove from heat and let eggs rest in water for 8 to 10 minutes. Remove eggs from pan and run under cold water. Cool and peel, discarding shells.

2. Mash avocado and eggs together until a textured and chunky in consistency. Add yogurt, mustard, lemon juice, and herbs. Season with salt and pepper to taste. Drizzle with olive oil.

3. Serve chilled or at room temperature. Transfer salad to a bowl if serving immediately or to an airtight container if saving for later. Store up to three days in the refrigerator.

Nutritional Information

Calories: 230 calories, Carbohydrates: 5g, Fat: 18g, Fiber: 2g, Protein: 13g, Saturated Fat: 5g, Sodium: 125mg, Sugar: 2g

Stovetop Eggplant Barley Paella

This recipe can be adapted for any season with whatever seasonal produce is on hand. Instead of eggplant, try zucchini in the summer or mushrooms in the fall.

Prep time: 75 minutes | Yield: Serves 4

Ingredients

- 2 cups pearl barley, washed

- 5 cups water

- 4 cups vegetable stock

- 1 sprig flat-leaf parsley, plus 3 tablespoons chopped

- Salt

- 2 tablespoons olive oil, plus more for drizzling

- 1 clove garlic, smashed and sliced

- 2 sprigs thyme, leaves stripped

- 2 shallots or 1 small onion, diced

- 1 poblano pepper, seeded, ribbed, and cut into thin strips

- 1 eggplant, cut into ¼-inch pieces

- ½ teaspoon ground cumin

- ½ teaspoon sweet smoked paprika

- 1 bay leaf

- ½ cup lemon juice

- 1 tablespoon chopped cilantro

Instructions

1. Thoroughly rinse fresh produce under warm running water for 20 seconds. Scrub to remove excess dirt.

2. Put barley in a pot with water, stock, parsley sprig, a good pinch of salt, and a drizzle of olive oil. Bring to a boil, then lower heat and simmer, covered, until barley is slightly undercooked, 25 to 30 minutes. (Barley will be cooked further later.)

3. While barley is cooking, heat 2 tablespoons olive oil over medium-high heat in a large frying pan. Add garlic and thyme and cook until garlic begins to brown. Add shallots and poblano pepper. Cook, stirring, until pepper softens and shallots start to caramelize. Add eggplant and 2 tablespoons chopped parsley.

4. Cook for a few minutes. Add cumin and paprika, cook for 1 minute, then add bay leaf and a pinch of salt. Mix well and cook until eggplant softens, about 7 to 10 minutes.

5. Add lemon juice and cook until the consistency is syrupy. Cover and reduce heat to low. Simmer for 10 minutes.

6. Remove parsley sprig and bay leaf from barley, then add semicooked barley, along with any cooking liquid left in the pot, to eggplant mixture.

7. Bring to a boil, then reduce heat and simmer, stirring occasionally, until barley is al dente, 10 to 15 minutes.

8. Stir in cilantro and remaining 1 tablespoon chopped parsley, heat through, and serve.

9. Paella should register 145 degrees Fahrenheit or higher using an instant-read thermometer placed in the middle of the dish.

Nutritional Information

Calories: 480 calories, Carbohydrates: 94g, Fat: 9g, Fiber: 21g, Protein: 12g, Saturated Fat: 1.5g, Sodium: 160mg, Sugar: 9g

Red Cabbage Slaw with Jicama and Mango

This cabbage salad has a tangy tropical twist with crunchy chopped jicama and juicy mango slices. Jicama is a root vegetable that is rich in vitamins and minerals. If you can't find it in stores, red bell pepper works well as a substitution.

Prep time: 20 minutes | Yield: Serves 8

Ingredients

- Cooking spray

- ½ cup pepitas or pumpkin seeds

- ½ cup sunflower seeds

- ½ head red cabbage, sliced thinly

- ½ jicama, peeled and chopped

- 1 mango (firm), sliced

- ¼ to ½ cup cilantro, chopped

- ½ cup pepitas or pumpkin seeds, toasted

- ½ cup sunflower seeds, toasted

- Juice from 2 limes

- ¼ cup rice wine vinegar

- 2 tablespoons honey

- ¼ cup extra-virgin olive oil

- Salt

Instructions

1. Thoroughly rinse fresh produce under warm running water for 20 seconds. Scrub to remove excess dirt.

2. Coat a skillet with cooking spray and toast seeds until brown, about 10 minutes.

3. Combine toasted seeds, cabbage, jicama, mango, cilantro, lime juice, vinegar, honey, and olive oil in a large bowl. Add salt to taste.

4. Serve immediately or transfer to an airtight container. Slaw can be stored up to 3 days in the refrigerator.

Nutritional Information

Calories: 210 calories, Carbohydrates: 14g, Fat: 15g, Fiber: 3g, Protein: 5g, Saturated Fat: 2.5g, Sodium: 170mg, Sugar: 9g

Edamame Hummus

This hummus is simply delicious. Packed with protein, edamame makes the perfect snack when you need a midday boost.

Prep time: 20 minutes | Yield: Serves 4-6

Ingredients

- 2 cups frozen shelled edamame

- 2 tablespoons tahini

- 2 cloves garlic, peeled

- 2 tablespoons olive oil

- 1 tablespoon cilantro leaves

- Juice of 2 lemons

- Salt and pepper

Instructions

1. Thoroughly rinse fresh produce under warm running water for 20 seconds.

2. Boil water in a medium saucepan. Add edamame and cook 1 to 2 minutes. Drain edamame and rinse under cold water to prevent it from cooking further.

3. Add cooked edamame, tahini, garlic, olive oil, cilantro, and lemon juice to a food processor or blender and pulse until smooth. Add salt and pepper to taste.

4. Serve immediately or transfer to an airtight container. Hummus can be stored up to 3 days in the refrigerator.

Nutritional Information

Calories: 150 calories, Carbohydrates: 10g, Fat: 9g, Fiber: 4g, Protein: 7g, Saturated Fat: 1g, Sodium: 20mg, Sugar: 1g

Kale and Wild Rice Casserole

Casseroles are a great make-ahead meal that can be portioned out for several days. If you're following the neutropenic diet, just be sure to follow guidelines for eating and storing leftovers. If you don't care for Gruyére, swap in your favorite pasteurized cheese.

Prep time: 95 minutes | Yield: Serves 8

Ingredients

- 2 large bunches kale, leaves removed from ribs and torn
- 1 cup water
- 4 tablespoons olive oil

- 1 pound cremini mushrooms, sliced

- 1 tablespoon butter

- 2 cloves garlic, minced or grated

- 2 tablespoons fresh thyme, chopped

- ¼ teaspoon nutmeg

- ¼ teaspoon salt, plus more for seasoning

- ½ teaspoon pepper, plus more for seasoning

- 4 tablespoons flour

- 1 cup pasteurized whole milk

- 1 cup chicken or vegetable broth

- ¼ cup coconut milk

- 4 cups cooked wild rice

- 1½ cups grated pasteurized Gruyére cheese

- 2 large sweet onions, sliced into thin rings

Instructions

1. Thoroughly rinse fresh produce under warm running water for 20 seconds. Scrub to remove excess dirt.

2. Preheat oven to 375 degrees. Grease a 2- or 3-quart casserole dish.

3. Heat a very large skillet over medium-high heat. Add kale and water, cover, and cook, stirring occasionally, until kale wilts, 10 to 15 minutes. Once kale is wilted and water is absorbed, remove skillet from heat and use tongs to remove kale to a plate. Set aside.

4. Using tongs, wipe skillet clean with paper towels. Return skillet to medium heat and add 2 tablespoons olive oil. Add mushrooms

in a single layer. Cook for 2 minutes without stirring. When bottoms are caramelized, use tongs to turn mushrooms once and season with ¼ teaspoon salt and ½ teaspoon pepper. Continue cooking without stirring for about 5 minutes.

5. Add butter to skillet and cook until it begins to brown. Reduce heat to low and add garlic, thyme, and nutmeg. Cook for about 10 seconds. Add cooked kale and toss to combine.

6. Sprinkle flour over kale mixture and cook for 1 minute. Add whole milk and broth and, stirring, bring to a boil. Reduce heat and

cook until thick, 2 to 3 minutes. Add cream and stir to combine.

7. Remove from heat and stir in rice. Pour mixture into prepared dish.

8. Using tongs, wipe skillet clean with paper towels. Add remaining 2 tablespoons olive oil and heat over medium-high. Add onions and salt and pepper to taste. Cook, stirring constantly, until onions begin to soften, about 5 minutes. Continue cooking until onions are golden brown, about 20 minutes.

9. Sprinkle half of the cheese over the casserole, then spread onions in an even layer. Top with remaining cheese. Bake until cheese is melted and onions are crispy, 20

to 25 minutes. Casserole should register 145 degrees Fahrenheit or higher using an instant-read thermometer in the middle of the dish.

Nutritional Information

Calories: 560 calories, Carbohydrates: 88g, Fat: 20g, Fiber: 8g, Protein: 18g, Saturated Fat: 8g, Sodium: 210mg, Sugar: 6g

Lentil Soup

Lentil soup is always a great option if you're having difficulties swallowing. Fresh rosemary and shallots gives this version its rich, comforting flavor.

Prep time: 50 minutes | Yield: Serves 4

Ingredients

- 2 tablespoons olive oil

- 2 shallots, minced

- 4 large carrots, washed, peeled, and sliced

- 2 cloves garlic, minced

- ½ teaspoon salt

- ½ teaspoon ground black pepper

- 2 sweet potatoes, washed, peeled, and diced

- 4 cups low-sodium vegetable or chicken broth

- 2 to 3 sprigs fresh rosemary, washed well

- 1 cup dry green or brown lentils, thoroughly rinsed and drained
- 2 cups chopped kale, very well washed

Instructions

1. Thoroughly rinse fresh produce under warm running water for 20 seconds. Scrub to remove excess dirt.

2. Heat a large pot over medium heat. Add olive oil, shallots, and carrots, and cook until carrots begin to soften, about 3 minutes. Add garlic and ¼ teaspoon each salt and pepper. Stir to combine, then cook until vegetables are tender, 4 to 5 minutes. Add sweet potatoes and remaining ¼ teaspoon

each salt and pepper. Stir and cook an additional 2 minutes.

3. Add broth and rosemary, then increase heat to medium high. Bring to a rolling simmer. Add lentils and stir to combine. Reduce heat to low and simmer, uncovered, until lentils and potatoes are tender, 15 to 20 minutes. Add kale, stir, and cover. Cook an additional 3 to 4 minutes to soften. Taste and adjust flavor by adding salt and pepper as needed.

4. To serve, soup should register 145 degrees Fahrenheit or higher using an instant-read thermometer in the middle of the dish.

Nutritional Information

Calories: 330 calories, Carbohydrates: 53g, Fat: 9g, Fiber: 12g, Protein: 14g, Saturated Fat: 1g, Sodium: 580mg, Sugar: 12g

Oven-Baked Chicken Fajitas

Serve this energizing dish with flour or corn tortillas or on a bed of brown rice. The portion for the Carbohydrate Controlled diet is two 6-inch tortillas or half a cup of brown rice.

Prep time: 20 minutes | Yield: Serves 4-6

Ingredients

- 1 tablespoon chili powder

- ½ tablespoon paprika

- ½ teaspoon onion powder

- ¼ teaspoon garlic powder

- ¼ teaspoon ground cumin

- ⅛ teaspoon cayenne pepper

- 1 teaspoon sugar

- ½ teaspoon salt

- 1 large onion, sliced in ¼-inch-wide strips

- 3 bell peppers, any color, sliced in ¼-inch-wide strips

- 1 pound boneless, skinless chicken breast, sliced in ¼-inch-wide strips

- 2 tablespoons vegetable oil

- Juice of half a lime

- 8 6-inch tortillas (flour or corn)

- ½ cup sour cream (optional)

- ¼ bunch fresh cilantro (optional)

Instructions

1. Thoroughly rinse fresh produce under warm running water for 20 seconds. Scrub to remove excess dirt.

2. Preheat oven to 400 degrees.

3. Mix the chili powder, paprika, onion powder, garlic powder, cumin, cayenne, sugar, and salt in a small bowl and set aside.

4. Spread onions and bell peppers in a 13x15 casserole dish or on a large rimmed baking

sheet. Top with sliced chicken. Drizzle oil over chicken and vegetables, then sprinkle seasoning mixture on top. Toss until combined. Bake 35 to 40 minutes, stirring once halfway through. Temperature of fajitas should be 165 degrees using an instant-read thermometer.

5. Sprinkle lime juice over fajitas and serve immediately with tortillas and, if using, sour cream and cilantro.

Nutritional Information

Calories: 300 calories, Carbohydrates: 12g, Fat: 12g, Fiber: 5g, Protein: 37g, Saturated Fat: 2g , Sodium: 270mg, Sugar: 6g

Portobello Mushroom Burgers

Portobello mushrooms make for juicy, tender veggie burgers that the whole family can enjoy.

Prep time: 45 minutes | Yield: Serves 8

Ingredients

- Cooking spray
- 3 tablespoons olive oil
- 1 small onion, finely chopped
- 6 cloves garlic, minced
- 1½ pounds portobello mushrooms, chopped
- 1 teaspoon red pepper flakes
- Salt and pepper

- 2½ cup bread crumbs (gluten free if desired)
- ½ cup grated carrots
- ⅓ cup green lentils, cooked
- 2 teaspoons dried parsley (optional)
- 2 teaspoons dried oregano (optional)
- 2 eggs, beaten

Instructions

1. Thoroughly rinse fresh produce under warm running water for 20 seconds. Scrub to remove excess dirt.
2. Preheat oven to 350 degrees. Coat a baking sheet with cooking spray.

3. Heat a large skillet over medium-low heat. Add 1 tablespoon olive oil and onion. Sauté onion until soft. Add garlic, mushrooms, and red pepper flakes. Season with salt and pepper to taste. Cook until mushrooms are brown, 5 to 8 minutes. Remove skillet from heat and transfer mushroom mixture to a large bowl to cool, at least 10 minutes.

4. Add panko, breadcrumbs, carrots, lentils, and herbs to mushroom mixture. Season to taste with salt and pepper. Add eggs and stir to combine. Divide mixture into 8 patties.

5. Reheat skillet over medium-low heat. Add the remaining 2 tablespoons olive oil. Cook

each patty until golden brown, 3 to 4 minutes per side.

6. Transfer patties to prepared baking sheet. Bake until cooked through, about 10 minutes. Internal temperature of patties should be 145 degrees using an instant-read thermometer. Serve warm.

Recipe Note:

If the burger mixture isn't sticking together, add more bread crumbs.

Nutritional Information

Calories:150 calories, Carbohydrates: 20g, Fat: 5g, Fiber: 3g, Protein: 6g, Saturated Fat: 1g, Sodium: 115mg, Sugar: 3g

Spaghetti Squash Casserole with Broccoli and Chicken

This protein-rich main course works with a variety of diets and can serve the whole family. Modify for a low-fiber diet by removing the broccoli.

Prep Time: 65 minutes | Yield: Serves 6

Ingredients

- 4 pounds spaghetti squash, halved lengthwise and seeded
- 2 tablespoons water
- 1 tablespoon extra-virgin olive oil
- 4 cloves garlic, minced
- 1 pound chicken breast, diced

96

- 2 cups broccoli florets, chopped

- ½ cup low-sodium chicken broth

- 1½ cups grated part-skim mozzarella cheese

- ½ cup grated Parmesan

- 1 teaspoon Italian seasoning

- 1 teaspoon salt

- ¼ teaspoon ground pepper

- ¼ cup panko bread crumbs

Instructions

1. Thoroughly rinse fresh produce under warm running water for 20 seconds. Scrub to remove excess dirt.

2. Position racks in upper and lower thirds of oven; preheat to 375 degrees.

3. Place squash cut-side down on a microwave-safe dish; add water and microwave on high until flesh is tender, 12 to 14 minutes. When cool, scrape flesh from rind in spaghetti like strands.

4. Heat olive oil in a skillet over medium-high heat. Add garlic and chicken; cook until chicken is browned on all sides. Add broccoli and broth, and cook for 2 minutes.

5. In a large bowl, toss shredded spaghetti squash and chicken mixture with ¾ cup mozzarella, 2 tablespoons Parmesan, Italian seasoning, salt, and pepper. Spread in an

oven-safe casserole dish. Sprinkle with remaining ¾ cup mozzarella and 6 tablespoons Parmesan; top with bread crumbs.

6. Bake on lower rack for 15 minutes. Move to upper rack and increase heat to 425 degrees. Bake until cheese browns, an additional 3 to 5 minutes.

7. Casserole should register 165 degrees Fahrenheit or higher using an instant-read thermometer placed in the middle of the dish.

Nutritional Information

Calories: 250calories, Carbohydrates: 14g, Fat: 11g, Fiber: 3g, Protein: 27g, Saturated Fat: 5g, Sodium: 690mg, Sugar: 3g

Tortilla Española

Tortilla española is a staple of Spanish cuisine. Heartily satisfying, it works well with many different diet types.

Prep time: 60 minutes | Yield: Serves 4

Ingredients

- ¼ cup extra-virgin olive oil
- 2 Yukon Gold potatoes, peeled and grated

- 1 medium yellow onion, thinly sliced

- Salt and pepper

- 8 eggs

Instructions

1. Preheat oven to 350 degrees.

2. In a 10-inch cast-iron skillet or other large oven-safe skillet, heat 2 tablespoons olive oil over medium heat. Add potatoes and onion. Season with salt. Cook, stirring occasionally, until onions are translucent. Set aside to cool; reserve skillet.

3. When potato mixture is cool, whisk eggs in a large bowl, then add potato mixture and

stir to combine. Season with salt and pepper.

4. Wipe skillet, add remaining 2 tablespoons olive oil, and return to medium heat. Add egg mixture. Cook, gently shaking skillet as egg begins to set. With a rubber spatula, scrape along the sides of the skillet to prevent sticking.

5. Once the sides are set, transfer skillet to oven. Bake about 15 minutes, making sure egg is cooked and not runny.

6. Internal temperature of tortilla española should be 160 degrees using an instant-read thermometer.

7. Allow tortilla to sit in skillet for 10 minutes before serving. Serve in wedges.

Nutritional Information

Calories: 290 calories, Carbohydrates: 6g, Fat: 22g, Fiber: 1g, Protein: 13g, Saturated Fat: 4g, Sodium: 230mg, Sugar: 4g

Banana Bread Muffins

Enjoy the moist goodness of fresh banana bread in the convenient shape of a muffin. If you like your muffins sweeter, try adding chocolate chips.

Prep time: 35 minutes | Yield: 12 Muffins

Ingredients

- 8 tablespoons (1 stick) butter, softened
- ¾ cup brown sugar
- ½ cup plain Greek yogurt
- 2 eggs
- 1 teaspoon vanilla
- 2 cups flour
- 1 teaspoon baking powder
- ¼ teaspoon baking soda
- ½ teaspoon cinnamon
- ¼ teaspoon ground ginger
- ½ teaspoon salt
- ½ cup mashed overripe banana

Instructions

1. Preheat oven to 350 degrees. Line a 12-cup muffin tin with muffin cups or parchment paper.

2. In a large bowl, cream butter with brown sugar, yogurt, eggs, and vanilla. Whisk in banana.

3. In a separate bowl, whisk flour, baking powder, baking soda, cinnamon, ginger, and salt.

4. Mix together the wet and dry ingredients in a large bowl until combined.

5. Divide batter evenly into prepared muffin tin.

6. Bake until golden and a toothpick inserted in the center of a muffin comes out clean, 20 to 25 minutes.

Nutritional Information

Calories: 210 calories, Carbohydrates: 29g, Fat: 9g, Fiber: 1g, Protein: 4g, Saturated Fat: 6g, Sodium: 180mg, Sugar: 14g

Mango Lassi

Mixing sweet ingredients with tart flavors, this balanced and delicious smoothie can help ease nausea. It's one the whole family will enjoy.

Prep time: 10 minutes | Yield: Serves 2

Ingredients

- 2 cups chopped mango

- ½ cup whole-milk yogurt

- ½ cup coconut milk or whole milk

- 1 teaspoon lime juice

- 1 teaspoon honey

- Pinch of cardamom

- 6 ice cubes

Instructions

1. Combine all ingredients in a blender. Pulse until smooth.

Nutritional Information

Calories: 260 calories, Carbohydrates: 32g, Fat: 15g, Fiber: 3g, Protein: 5g, Saturated Fat: 12g, Sodium: 35mg, Sugar: 28g

Cantaloupe and Mint Granita

Originating in Sicily, granitas are similar to Italian ice. They're also heart healthier than ice cream and so easy to make. This refreshing version combines the creamy sweetness of cantaloupe with the tang of lime and mint.

Prep Time: 35 minutes | Cool time: 8 hours | Yield: Serves 10-12

Ingredients

- 2 cups water

- 1 cup sugar, or more to taste

- 1¼ cup fresh mint leaves

- 1 cantaloupe, peeled, seeded, and chopped

- 3 tablespoons lime juice

Instructions

2. Thoroughly rinse fresh produce under warm running water for 20 seconds. Scrub to remove excess dirt.

3. In a small saucepan, combine the water, 1 cup sugar, and 1 cup mint leaves. Bring to a boil over medium heat. Reduce heat and simmer, stirring occasionally, until sugar has

dissolved, about 5 minutes. Remove pan from heat and set aside to cool, about 20 minutes. Pour cooled syrup through a strainer to remove mint leaves.

4. In a blender, puree the strained syrup, cantaloupe, and lime juice until smooth, then taste. To sweeten more, add 1 tablespoon sugar at a time and blend; taste and repeat until desired flavor is reached. Add remaining mint leaves and blend until finely chopped.

5. Pour the mixture into a 9x13 glass baking dish and freeze, at least 8 hours or overnight.

6. Using the tines of a fork, scrape the granita to the desired texture and serve in chilled bowls.

Recipe Note

Letting the granita sit on the counter for 5 to 10 minutes makes it smoother and easier to swallow.

Nutritional Information

Calories: 90 calories, Carbohydrates: 22g, Fat: 0g, Fiber: 1g, Protein: 1g, Saturated Fat: 0g, Sodium: 10mg, Sugar: 21g

TAKEAWAY

The neutropenic diet incorporates dietary changes to help prevent you from consuming harmful bacteria in foods and beverages. This diet is specifically meant for people with neutropenia, who are always advised to follow the FDA's food safety guidelines. It's also implemented among those with cancer and weakened immune systems.

Though some institutions incorporate this diet into medical treatment plans, more research is needed to demonstrate its effectiveness. Traditional treatment methods shouldn't be ignored. Prior to participating in a new diet, discuss your options and risks with your doctor.

Made in the USA
Las Vegas, NV
13 September 2024